COMPREHENSIVE CURRICULUM-BASED TRAINING FOR YOUNG COMPETITIVE SWIMMERS

RAPOLAS JANONIS

© Copyright 2024 - Coachology LLC. All rights reserved.

It is not legal to reproduce, duplicate, or transmit any part of this document in either electronic means or in printed format. Recording of this publication is strictly prohibited and any storage of this document is not allowed unless with written permission from the publisher except for the use of brief quotations in a book review.

This book or any portion thereof may not be reproduced or used in any manner whatsoever without the express written permission of the publisher except for the use of brief quotations in a book review.

First edition, 2024.

www.coachology.info

CONTENTS

Introduction	vii

1. CURRICULUM-BASED TRAINING FOR YOUNG SWIMMERS — 1
The Spiral Curriculum: Building Blocks of Learning — 2
Deliberate Practice: The Path to Mastery — 6
The Journey to Excellence — 10

2. DESIGNING A SWIM SEASON — 13
Structuring the Training Season — 14
Breaking Down the Training Block — 15
Coaching Benefits — 19
Equitable Time Allocation for All Competitive Events — 20
Benefits of Implementing Curriculum-Based Training Season Design — 23

3. STRUCTURING EFFECTIVE SWIM PRACTICES — 25
Warm-Up: Establishing Discipline and Focus — 25
The Training Sets in Curriculum-Based Training — 27
The Role of Relays in Curriculum-Based Training — 29
Benefits of Implementing Curriculum-Based Training for Young Swimmers — 33

4. TRAINING SET STRUCTURE — 37
Summary and Coaches' Benefits of Curriculum-Based Training Sets — 42

5. A COMPREHENSIVE APPROACH TO SKILL DEVELOPMENT IN CURRICULUM-BASED TRAINING — 46
Implementation in Curriculum-Based Training — 50
Building Mastery Through Stroke Development — 52

6. PSYCHOLOGY AND COMPETITION — 55
Reducing Anxiety — 56
Peer Pressure — 57
Maintaining Motivation — 60
Power of Words — 61

Psychology of Words in Curriculum-Based Training	63
Long-Term Benefits	64
Conclusion	67
About the Author	71
References	73

To My Coach, Gintautas Bartkus,

You ignited a fire within me that has fueled my passion for swimming and shaped me into the athlete and person I am today. Your unwavering dedication, steadfast support, and expert guidance have been the cornerstone of my success both in and out of the pool.

Your belief in me never wavered, even when I doubted myself. Your words of encouragement and wisdom pushed me to strive for greatness and never settle for mediocrity. You saw my potential when I could not see it in myself, and for that, I am forever grateful. You taught me the value of hard work, discipline, and perseverance. Your relentless pursuit of excellence inspired me to push beyond my limits and achieve things I never thought possible. Your coaching provided valuable guidance that extended beyond just improving my swimming; it also served as a source of mentorship that helped me enhance my personal growth both within and outside the pool.

I am proud to have had you as my coach, mentor, and friend. Your impact on my life is immeasurable, and I will carry the lessons you have taught me for the rest of my days. Thank you for being the guiding light in my swimming journey, for believing in me when no one else did, and for helping me become the best version of myself.

With heartfelt gratitude and admiration,

Rapolas Janonis

INTRODUCTION

The *Comprehensive Curriculum-Based Training for Young Competitive Swimmers* presents a novel approach that recognizes swimmers as continuous learners in a dynamic process of growth and improvement. Thus, this book serves as an introduction to the Curriculum-Based Training method and advocates for a focus on steady and continual improvement rather than striving for perfection. Drawing on the research of esteemed scholars such as Dr. Jerome S. Bruner and Dr. Anders Ericsson, it presents a methodology designed to enhance learning and facilitate development.

As the title suggests, this book provides useful ideas to coach young swimmers utilizing a blend of progressive skills and mental training that are all based on the principles of progressive learning, progressive skill acquisition, and mental preparedness for competition. This publication prepares swimmers for the effective acquisition of proper stroke mechanics, as well as effective racing skills. As a combination of theory and training practice, *Comprehensive Curriculum-Based Training for Young Competitive Swimmers* is a powerful method for helping coaches and young swimmers understand the challenges involved and find ways to develop themselves in the world of competitive swimming.

My approach is based on the belief that swimmers are learners in a process of development. I understand that every swimmer is at a different level of learning, and their technical skills are always changing and developing. Whenever I coach someone, I don't take the view that the swimmer requires fixing or that there's something wrong with them, but rather, they are in a constant process of learning and growing.

I recognize the dynamic nature of physical and mental changes that impact athletes and embrace the technical and intangible elements that, blended together, can create a remarkable young swimmer. I strive to create a supportive and nurturing environment that fosters a mindset of learning and improvement. By shifting the focus from perceived shortcomings to a mindset of growth and progress, my aim is to empower swimmers to embrace the journey, celebrate their achievements, and keep pushing toward their full potential.

The Curriculum-Based Training method was conceptualized with a holistic perspective on young competitive swimmers. It takes into account not only their physical attributes but also their psychological and developmental aspects. With a philosophy centered on the belief that athletes are always progressing and growing rather than just needing correction, this method has evolved over nearly two decades. Instead of focusing on identifying flaws, the approach regards each swimmer as being on a unique developmental journey with continual advancement in mind.

While some approaches may prioritize fixing specific elements of a swimmer's performance, this method prioritizes the continual refinement of stroke mechanics and racing skills through motor learning processes embedded in the brain. My own background includes advanced graduate studies in swimming research with a principle of specificity, as well as personal swimming experiences that have ranged over twenty years and taken me from Lithuania to the United States and through diverse coaching roles in different competitive environments. Drawing inspiration from Dr. Jerome S. Bruner's spiral curriculum model, this approach acknowledges and accommodates the distinctive characteristics and needs of young swimmers.

CHAPTER 1
CURRICULUM-BASED TRAINING FOR YOUNG SWIMMERS

In the thrilling, fast-paced world of competitive swimming, achieving success involves far more than pure talent and grit. Many people have potential talent, but too often, their latent abilities aren't fully developed due to inadequate training methods. What is required is a structured approach to developing skills that are not only physical but also psychological.

Enter the Curriculum-Based Training method—the method designed with great care to help young swimmers reach their highest possible level by implementing the principles of educational psychology and deliberate practice.

The Curriculum-Based Training method is underpinned by two foundational theories: Dr. Jerome S. Bruner's spiral curriculum model and Dr. Anders Ericsson's principles of deliberate practice. These theories coalesce into a comprehensive strategy aimed at facilitating young swimmers' progression through various stages of learning while encouraging self-education and self-improvement that inherently promote cognitive development.

THE SPIRAL CURRICULUM: BUILDING BLOCKS OF LEARNING

The concept of the spiral curriculum, introduced by cognitive psychology pioneer Dr. Jerome S. Bruner in the 1960s, is a transformative approach to education. This model emphasizes structuring learning experiences so that students revisit the same fundamental concepts repeatedly, each time encountering them at a progressively higher level of difficulty. This iterative learning process ensures that foundational skills are not only learned but deeply ingrained and continually refined.

In the context of training young swimmers, the spiral curriculum means that fundamental movements are taught from the very beginning. These movements are not simply repeated but are revisited and enhanced over time. For example, a young swimmer might start by learning the basic butterfly stroke. Initially, the focus might be on basic body position and the rudimentary coordination of arm and leg movements. As the swimmer's proficiency increases, they revisit the stroke during the practice sessions, each time incorporating more complex elements such as efficient breathing patterns, precise arm movements, and optimized speed.

This repeated and layered approach builds a robust foundation while simultaneously enhancing the swimmer's skills. Every time they go back to each stroke, it is an opportunity for improvement and learning. The swimmer becomes more fine-tuned with each attempt they make, thus promoting efficiency in the manner in which they swim.

In addition, the organization of the curriculum in spirals helps young swimmers to recapitulate the previous learning and develop the cognitive connections for new, more complicated information. This method is appropriate to the development of competitive skills because one has to learn the fundamental stroke skills before mastering the other complex mechanics. To the young swimmers, it comes down to the fact that consistent training sessions with a focus on gradual improvement are crucial in mastering the fundamental competitive skills.

It also helps in developing a positive attitude in young swimmers known as growth mindset. Thus, while focusing on the process of performance enhancement and knowing that there is always room for improvement and learning, young swimmers become more perseverant and committed to learning —and this approach often continues throughout their lives. They are able to understand that becoming an expert is not a one day affair; it is achieved through hard work and step by step determination.

The spiral curriculum is flexible and the needs of any one swimmer can be incorporated. Revisitation of the fundamental skill work can be planned to overcome certain deficiencies or to elaborate on certain assets. This implies that each swimmer is carefully guided to improve at his or her own rate and level of capacity, which is very important in competitive swimming.

Summing up, the spiral curriculum is all about building an effective learning environment that is constantly developing and changing. It understands that acquiring skills is not a linear process; on the contrary, it is a recursive process that requires constant practice and complexity in the way it is taught. For young swimmers, this results in a more efficient and complete training process that provides not only the foundation of the proper stroke mechanics but also the gradual improvement of skills, as well as cognitive abilities. By the use of the spiral curriculum, young swimmers are well equipped to attain excellence in water because training is based on the progression of the swimmer's ability and knowledge.

Benefits of Curriculum-Based Training

The innovative Curriculum-Based Training method for young swimmers offers numerous benefits. Firstly, it helps improve overall performance by providing a structured and strategic approach to training that optimizes skill development. By following a carefully designed curriculum, swimmers can track their progress, set goals, and work towards achieving consistent improvement in their abilities.

This method also facilitates the improvement of competitive stroke mechanics by starting with foundational principles and gradually increasing levels of complexity. Through diligent practice, young swimmers can enhance their overall efficiency in the water, ultimately leading to improved acquisition of competitive skills.

Fostering Self-Awareness and Self-Correction

Self-awareness is a fundamental component of the Curriculum-Based Training approach, which is designed to support young swimmers in developing a heightened sense of their body in the water. This fosters an independent understanding of their strengths and areas for improvement, empowering them to make self-adjustments and enhance their overall performance.

The advantages of self-awareness transcend physical abilities and talents, encompassing cognitive growth through activities that emphasize self-regulation. Participation in such activities has been shown to promote the development of gray matter in the brain. Young swimmers inevitably benefit from enhanced cognitive development as they evaluate and refine their skills.

Furthermore, the process of self-correction is essential in fostering resilience and adaptability in young swimmers. By identifying and rectifying mistakes or shortcomings in their swimming strokes, turns, and dives, they can make required adjustments.

The integration of the Curriculum-Based Training method promotes self-awareness and individual growth, leading to improved skill acquisition. This approach emphasizes a commitment to continuous improvement, perceiving challenges as chances for growth and refinement rather than obstacles.

Systematic and Structured Training

The Curriculum-Based Training approach stands out for its systematic and organized methodology, which is essential for fostering both technical proficiency and mental resilience in young swimmers. This approach ensures that every aspect of training is carefully planned and executed, maximizing the benefits for each swimmer.

The structured nature of The Curriculum-Based Training also helps instill a sense of discipline in young swimmers. Training sessions are conducted in a highly organized manner, with clear objectives and routines. This disciplined approach is crucial in a sport that demands precision and consistency. By training in a structured environment, young swimmers learn to approach their practice sessions with the seriousness and commitment that competitive swimming requires. This disciplined atmosphere enhances technical skills and fosters a strong work ethic and a sense of responsibility.

Within the Curriculum-Based Training framework, coaches serve a multifaceted role as both mentors and motivators. In their capacity as mentors, they offer essential feedback to swimmers, aiding in the identification of areas for adjustment and providing guidance for improvement. This feedback is integral for continuous skill refinement and overall progress. As motivators, coaches provide the necessary encouragement and inspiration to keep young swimmers committed and enthusiastic about their training regimen. This dual role is particularly significant in light of the inevitable challenges and setbacks that arise in any training program. Coaches adept at inspiring and motivating their swimmers play a pivotal role in helping them navigate obstacles and sustain their focus and determination.

The structured approach of Curriculum-Based Training plays a crucial role in effectively managing the training workload. Training sessions are methodically designed to incrementally enhance both intensity and complexity, thereby enabling young swimmers to develop their skills steadily. This systematic progression serves as a safeguard against burnout and overtraining, promoting sustainable performance in the long run. Coaches maintain diligent supervision over the swimmers' progress, fine-tuning the training regimen as necessary to ensure consistent advancement while mitigating the risks of injury and exhaustion.

DELIBERATE PRACTICE: THE PATH TO MASTERY

The concept of deliberate practice emphasizes that not *all* practice is equal. Simply spending hours swimming in the pool does not guarantee improvement in a swimmer's performance. Deliberate practice involves setting specific goals, seeking feedback, and pushing yourself to the limits of your ability. By adhering to this systematic and intentional approach, young swimmers are motivated to consistently strive for improvement.

The principle of deliberate practice is founded on the premise that advancement arises not solely from mere repetition, but from concentrated and purposeful interaction with a particular skill. In the context of swimming, this principle dictates that merely going through the motions in the pool is insufficient for substantial development. By establishing precise and attainable objectives, swimmers can channel their energy towards refining specific elements of their swimming that are in need of enhancement. This tailored strategy not only guarantees the efficient use of practice time but also sustains young swimmers' motivation and involvement by offering tangible goals to pursue.

Receiving feedback is an essential part of deliberate practice for improving swimming skills. Constructive criticism from coaches, peers, or performance data provides valuable insights into a swimmer's strengths and weaknesses. This feedback helps young swimmers achieve continuous refinement of their skills. Identifying areas that require focused efforts and making necessary adjustments is essential for improvement. Accepting feedback cultivates a mentality of constant learning and growth. This encourages young swimmers to recognize that there are always opportunities for improvement.

One fundamental principle of deliberate practice lies in the dedicated pursuit of pushing one's abilities to the utmost limit, as distinct from mere passive repetition. By consistently embracing challenges and stepping outside their comfort zones, aspiring young swimmers can accelerate their learning curve and elevate their skillset.

This ethos of pushing boundaries and striving for excellence cultivates a strong work ethic and resilience while also instilling discipline and perseverance in young swimmers. By consistently applying deliberate practice, swimmers can fully immerse themselves in the continuous pursuit of improvement.

Implementing Deliberate Practice in Training

To effectively incorporate deliberate practice in training, it is essential to focus on key elements such as establishing specific goals, providing feedback, and encouraging self-reflection. These components play a crucial role in shaping a young swimmer's skill acquisition and the fostering of improvement.

- **Goal Setting:** Deliberate practice begins with the clear setting of goals and objectives. These goals should be specific, measurable, achievable, and relevant. Establishing goals in collaboration with the swimmer is essential, as it fosters ownership and commitment to the training process. Goals should combine short-term and long-term perspectives to provide immediate targets for improvement and a broader vision for future achievements. Short-term goals might include refining a specific stroke or improving competitive turns over a few weeks, while long-term goals could involve achieving a personal best at an upcoming competition or qualifying for a major event.

- **Focused Practice:** Each training session should be planned with a clear objective, focusing on enhancing a specific skill set. This precise approach guarantees that swimmers are investing their time and energy into mastering fundamental components crucial for their advancement. For instance, if a training session is focused on improving streamline, it will be strategically designed to maximize the swimmers' proficiency in this aspect. During the session, there is a focus on utilizing streamline effectively in training sets, turns, and dives. By dedicating practice time to specific skills, swimmers can achieve significant improvements in targeted areas, leading to a specific skill enhancement.

- **Immediate Feedback:** Feedback is a vital component of deliberate practice, providing young swimmers with the information they need to understand their performance and make necessary adjustments. Coaches should offer immediate, specific feedback during and after practice sessions. This feedback helps swimmers recognize what they are doing correctly and identify areas that need improvement. For example, if a swimmer's stroke needs refinement, the coach can provide real-time corrections and suggestions to help young swimmers make adjustments. Consistent, constructive feedback accelerates learning and ensures that swimmers are always aware of their progress and areas for improvement.

- **Challenging Tasks:** Intentional practice for young swimmers entails providing tasks that push their current limits, encouraging them to tackle more advanced challenges. This can include introducing new, complex skills or increasing the difficulty of existing tasks. For instance, coaches may incorporate extra technical elements or introduce fresh concepts. These demanding tasks are crucial for progress, as they compel young swimmers to adjust and cultivate new abilities, resulting in ongoing enhancements.

- **Reflection and Adaptation:** Reflection and adaptation play a pivotal role in the sustained growth and achievement of young swimmers. It is imperative for them to assess their performance, carefully analyze feedback, and effectively implement necessary adjustments. Engaging in reflective learning empowers young swimmers to cultivate self-awareness and active participation in their training regimen. Following each practice session or competition, swimmers are encouraged to evaluate their strengths, weaknesses, and areas for enhancement. This reflective practice enables swimmers to internalize valuable insights and integrate them into their future training endeavors, thereby fostering a culture of ongoing progression.

- **Integrating All Elements:** To effectively integrate these elements into a cohesive training program, coaches should follow a structured approach. Begin each training cycle by setting clear, attainable goals with the young swimmer. Design practice sessions that focus on specific skills, ensuring each session has a clear objective. Provide immediate, actionable feedback throughout the training process, and regularly challenge young swimmers with tasks that stretch their abilities. Encourage swimmers to reflect on their performance and adapt based on their reflections and the feedback they've received (Busch, 2024).

THE JOURNEY TO EXCELLENCE

My extensive background in swimming dates back many years, encompassing roles as both a competitive swimmer, swimming instructor, and coach. Through these various experiences, I have gained valuable insights into the sport from both an athlete's and a coach's perspective. My initial experience in designing a curriculum for a learn-to-swim program laid the foundation for meticulous planning and execution in swim education.

The endeavor to establish a comprehensive learn-to-swim program aimed to surpass traditional swimming education methods. The intention was to develop a program that not only imparts basic swimming skills to children but also nurtures a passion for continual improvement in their swimming abilities.

My pursuit extended beyond instructing young swimmers, as I harbored a keen interest in understanding the cognitive processes involved in their learning experiences. This drive has propelled me to enhance their motor learning abilities. Subsequently, my endeavor has evolved towards devising an interdisciplinary curriculum that not only focuses on the physical aspects of swimming but also incorporates elements that cater to the cognitive and psychological development of the child.

Transition to Coaching

After my swimming competition years were over, I transitioned to the profession of full-time swimming coach. This shift allowed me to channel my efforts and learning toward helping others reach their potential in the pool. I found great satisfaction in applying my knowledge and experience to guide young swimmers, and this new chapter in my life became a profound learning journey in itself.

It was during this time that I was privileged to be tutored by Dr. Ben Zhou, a distinguished expert in Exercise Science, specifically in the areas of aerobic capacity and fitness tests. Under Dr. Zhou's mentorship, I developed a deeper understanding of the scientific principles underlying athletic performance. This mentorship was invaluable as I began to craft training programs designed to enhance both the physical and mental aspects of swimming performance. Dr. Zhou's insights into the physiological and psychological demands of swimming provided a solid foundation for my coaching methodologies.

Inspired by Dr. Zhou's lectures, I felt motivated to further my educational objectives and decided to pursue a major in kinesiology. This decision was driven by a desire to deepen my understanding of the science of exercise and to integrate this knowledge into my coaching practice. Dr. Zhou played a significant role in shaping my worldview regarding the intricate link between the body and the mind. His teachings emphasized the importance of a holistic approach to training, one that considers the athlete's overall well-being rather than focusing solely on physical performance.

This holistic perspective became a cornerstone of my coaching philosophy. I adopted the principle of training for well-being, which targets the enhancement of both a swimmer's physical and psychological potential. This approach involves incorporating mental conditioning techniques, such as goal setting, visualization, and stress management, into the training regimen. By fostering a positive and supportive environment, I aim to help swimmers build resilience, confidence, and a growth-oriented mindset.

My transition to coaching has been a deeply rewarding experience. It's allowed me to combine my passion for swimming with my commitment to helping others achieve their best. By integrating scientific knowledge with practical coaching techniques, I aim to inspire young swimmers to pursue excellence and develop a lifelong love for the sport. Through my work, I hope to make a lasting impact on the lives of the athletes I coach, guiding them toward success in the pool and beyond.

Advanced Studies and Specialization

Earning a graduate degree in kinesiology has equipped me with a specialized focus on swimming coaching, centered on the principles of sports psychology and specificity. Through rigorous study and practical application, I have developed expertise in designing training programs that address both the physical development and motor learning capabilities of young swimmers.

During my tenure as a graduate student and swimming coach, I leveraged my academic knowledge to develop and implement the Curriculum-Based Training methodology at the pool. This innovative approach focused on holistic development, integrating physical, cognitive, and behavioral training for young swimmers.

By adhering to these principles, coaches will enhance their capacity to cultivate a new cohort of young swimmers who possess the aptitude to excel not only in the pool but also in various facets of life.

CHAPTER 2
DESIGNING A SWIM SEASON

The journey to success in competitive swimming starts with a properly planned training season. Young swimmers need to have a carefully structured curriculum to enhance their performance and meet the set objectives. The Curriculum-Based Training method provides a clear structure based on educational psychology and deliberate practice for swimmers' development. This chapter provides a deeper look into the components of structuring a training season, especially the aspect of equal time distribution across all competitive events.

The Curriculum-Based Training method for young competitive swimmers has a carefully planned swim season that aims to enhance their skills and abilities thoroughly. The season is divided into four-week blocks, with each week dedicated to one essential element crucial for swimming success: streamline, head/body position, breathing mechanics, and pull phase. This structured approach enables young swimmers to deeply explore and improve each element, ultimately refining their stroke, turn, and dive mechanics.

Furthermore, it is essential to highlight the importance of deliberate practice when designing a successful swim season. This principle guarantees that focus is equally allocated to all competitive events according to each age group. Such an approach to a specific skill development guarantees that young swimmers have the chance to shine in every aspect of competitive swimming, rather than being limited to mastering a single stroke or event. Implementing a well-rounded training program that covers all competitive events helps prevent young swimmers from becoming overly specialized, which can lead to fatigue and hinder their overall progress.

It is crucial for young swimmers to distribute their training time effectively across all competitive events to prevent burnout and encourage overall development. The Curriculum-Based Training season is designed to enhance a diverse range of skills and achieve proficiency in every event, equipping young swimmers with the essential abilities for success and a lasting love for the sport. This strategy prioritizes well-rounded skill building and comprehensive training, setting young swimmers up to fully realize their potential in their swimming endeavors.

STRUCTURING THE TRAINING SEASON

The Curriculum-Based Training method provides a holistic approach to training young competitive swimmers by focusing on fundamental aspects of swimming in a systematic manner. By dividing the swim season into four-week blocks, the method ensures that each vital element is given ample attention and time for improvement. This deliberate structure allows young swimmers to gradually build upon their skills and abilities, setting a strong foundation for long-term success in the sport. By dedicating each week to a specific aspect such as streamline, head/body position, breathing mechanics, and pull phase, swimmers can develop a deep understanding of the technical nuances of each component, leading to more refined stroke mechanics and increased efficiency in the water.

Additionally, the attention to detail in the Curriculum-Based Training method encourages young swimmers to focus on quality over quantity. By emphasizing the importance of mastering individual elements before moving on to more complex skills, swimmers can develop a strong technical foundation that will serve them well in their competitive endeavors. This approach not only enhances their swimming abilities but also reduces the risk of injury by ensuring that proper stroke mechanics are in place before progressing to more advanced elements. As a result, swimmers are better equipped to excel in races and handle the physical demands of competitive swimming with confidence and proficiency.

Moreover, the Curriculum-Based Training method fosters a sense of discipline and dedication in young swimmers as they work toward mastering the essential fundamentals of swimming. By following a structured training season and diligently focusing on perfecting different elements each week, young swimmers learn valuable lessons in perseverance and goal-setting. This design instills a mindset of continuous improvement and growth, encouraging young swimmers to strive for excellence in all aspects of their swimming performance. Ultimately, the carefully planned swim season not only enhances the physical skills of young competitive swimmers but also cultivates important life skills such as self-discipline, resilience, and goal achievement.

BREAKING DOWN THE TRAINING BLOCK

Week One: Streamline

In every training block of the Curriculum-Based Training season, a strong emphasis is placed on the importance of streamline during the first week. Developing a strong foundation in streamline from the outset can greatly improve the overall swimming proficiency, particularly in aspects such as turns and dives. Not only does proper streamline reduce drag, but it also enables swimmers to optimize their energy consumption, thus enhancing their swimming efficiency.

By emphasizing streamlined positioning at the beginning of each training block, young swimmers have the opportunity to significantly enhance their speed and overall skills. It is vital to understand that maintaining a streamlined position is not limited to the initial push off the wall; rather, it should be a continuous focus throughout every aspect of their swimming.

In the realm of competitive swimming, the maintenance of streamline is imperative for achieving success in all strokes. In a sport that hinges on the precision of timing, the capacity to uphold a streamlined position can substantially influence the outcome, determining victory or defeat.

Week Two: Head and Body Position

During the second week of each training block, the Curriculum-Based Training places significant emphasis on enhancing head and body positions in all swimming strokes. This targeted focus aligns with the principle of purposeful practice, as advocated by Dr. Ericsson, encouraging concentrated and deliberate efforts in specific areas to drive improvement. By meticulously addressing the nuances of head and body positioning, swimmers can enhance their technical proficiency and biomechanical efficiency across various strokes. This systematic approach enables young swimmers to make gradual progress in their performance, facilitating consistent development and advancement.

It is paramount to emphasize the significance of maintaining proper head and body positioning in swimming, particularly for the developmental advancement of young swimmers. A precise alignment of the head and body not only boosts hydrodynamics but also reduces water resistance, facilitating enhanced speed and efficiency. Additionally, accurate positioning is crucial for activating core muscle groups, leading to increased power generation and propulsion. By ingraining these fundamental principles in young swimmers early on, a solid foundation for their swimming skills can be established.

Furthermore, the proficiency in head and body positioning throughout all swimming strokes is essential for developing enhanced body awareness and coordination in young swimmers. Utilizing a structured Curriculum-Based Training method allows swimmers to concentrate on these precise components, resulting in a deeper comprehension of their movements in the water and the subtle modifications that can greatly influence their performance.

Week Three: Breathing Mechanics

The utilization of the Curriculum-Based Training method is crucial in emphasizing the significance of correct breathing mechanics in swimming. By incorporating a tailored focus on developing appropriate breathing mechanics during training sessions, young swimmers can enhance their ability to maintain a consistent rhythm and reduce fatigue levels. The systematic approach of this method designates every third week of the training block for an intensive concentration on perfecting efficient breathing patterns.

Effective breathing mechanics are essential for young swimmers as they aim to optimize oxygen intake and sustain their performance. Proficient breathing ensures a consistent flow of oxygen to the muscles, reducing early fatigue, and it also plays a vital role in enhancing race performance.

Moreover, the Curriculum-Based Training acknowledges the comprehensive benefits of effective breathing mechanics for young swimmers. In addition to the physical advantages, developing proficiency in proper breathing enhances psychological well-being by elevating performance levels, instilling confidence, and fostering mental acuity and resilience. This holistic methodology not only enhances training results but also empowers young swimmers with the skills needed to adeptly handle stress and elevate their competitive prowess.

Week Four: Pull Phase

In the final week of each training block utilizing the Curriculum-Based Training, there is a strategic emphasis placed on refining the pull phase of each competitive swimming stroke. This period is dedicated to providing young swimmers with the opportunity to enhance their efficiency in this essential component of their strokes. By focusing in on the pull phase, swimmers can concentrate on developing the necessary power and propulsion required to effectively navigate through the water. This targeted focus enables young swimmers to fine-tune their movements and build specific strength.

By integrating the deliberate practice principle into the training, young swimmers are able to participate in focused and systematic practice sessions designed to enhance their skills. By dissecting the pull phase into smaller segments, swimmers can pinpoint and address specific areas requiring enhancement in a methodical manner. This approach of targeted and repetitive practice has the potential to yield substantial improvements in efficiency.

Enhancing efficiency in the pull phase of each stroke is paramount for optimizing the physical abilities of young swimmers, while also yielding psychological advantages. As swimmers witness tangible advancements in their stroke efficiency and speed during training sessions, their confidence in their capabilities is bolstered, cultivating a constructive mindset towards their athletic development. Setting precise objectives pertaining to the pull phase and successfully attaining them through deliberate practice instills a profound sense of achievement and drive in young swimmers, thereby fostering heightened motivation and performance enhancement during competitive events.

COACHING BENEFITS

The Curriculum-Based Training method offers numerous benefits for coaches working with young competitive swimmers. Firstly, the systematic approach of dividing the swim season into four-week blocks allows coaches to plan and structure training sessions with a clear focus on fundamental aspects of swimming. This structured approach helps coaches ensure that each vital element, such as streamline, head/body position, breathing mechanics, and pull phase, is thoroughly addressed and improved upon. By having a well-thought-out plan in place, coaches can track the progress of swimmers more effectively and tailor their coaching strategies to meet the specific needs of each individual swimmer.

Secondly, the emphasis on quality over quantity in the Curriculum-Based Training season design encourages coaches to prioritize technical mastery and skill development. By dedicating specific weeks to refining particular aspects of swimming, coaches can help young swimmers build a strong technical foundation before progressing to more advanced skills. This focus on meticulous attention to detail not only enhances the swimming abilities of young athletes but also reduces the risk of injury by ensuring that proper stroke mechanics are in place. Coaches can use this approach to instill a culture of precision and excellence in their swimmers, setting them up for success in competitive races and long-term growth in the sport.

Furthermore, the Curriculum-Based Training planned season fosters a sense of discipline and dedication in young swimmers, which can be attributed to the structured and goal-oriented nature of the training program. Coaches can leverage this approach to teach valuable life skills such as self-discipline, resilience, and goal achievement to their athletes. By guiding young swimmers through a carefully planned training season that focuses on continuous improvement and growth, coaches can help instill a mindset of perseverance and excellence in their athletes. This holistic development not only benefits young swimmers in their athletic pursuits but also equips them with essential life skills that extend beyond the pool.

EQUITABLE TIME ALLOCATION FOR ALL COMPETITIVE EVENTS

The equitable allocation of time across competitive events is vital in swim training for young competitive swimmers. This method ensures comprehensive coverage of essential skills and facilitates the development of a well-structured training schedule, both of which are crucial for a young swimmer's competitive edge in the future. Therefore, it is imperative to further elaborate on the significance of distributing training time evenly among all competitive events.

Comprehensive Skill Development

First and foremost, the equitable allocation of time across various competitive events in swim training ensures that young swimmers develop a well-rounded skill set. Each competitive event in swimming demands a different skill set, strengths, and strategies. By dedicating an equal amount of time to each event throughout the season, swimmers can focus on improving their proficiency in all aspects of their performance. This approach not only cultivates versatility but also helps young swimmers discover their strengths and weaknesses in different events, allowing them to fine-tune their skills and maximize their potential.

Moreover, distributing training time evenly among all competitive events empowers swimmers to create a well-structured and balanced training schedule. By allocating time strategically to different events, coaches and swimmers can plan specific training sets tailored to the requirements of each competitive event. This systematic and organized approach not only enhances the effectiveness of training sessions but also prevents overtraining in specific events, reducing the risk of burnout or injuries. A well-structured training schedule ensures that young swimmers progress steadily in all events, building a strong foundation for long-term success in competitive swimming.

Furthermore, the equitable allocation of time among competitive events in swim training is essential for nurturing a young swimmer's competitive edge in the future. Consistent and balanced training across all events instills discipline, determination, and mental fortitude in swimmers, preparing them for the challenges of competitive swimming. It also fosters a sense of adaptability and resilience, enabling swimmers to face various competitive scenarios with confidence and versatility. Ultimately, by emphasizing the importance of distributing training time evenly among all competitive events, coaches and swimmers can lay a solid groundwork for continuous improvement, growth, and success in competitive swimming.

Prevention of Over-Specialization

Balancing training time across all competitive events is not only important for preventing overloading but also for fostering a well-rounded development in young swimmers. By avoiding over-specialization, coaches can help athletes explore different strokes and distances, thereby broadening their skill sets and maintaining their passion for the sport. Diversifying training also minimizes the risk of burnout and injuries, allowing swimmers to enjoy a longer and healthier career in the pool.

In the delicate phase of physical development that young swimmers are in, it's crucial for coaches to understand the need for a holistic approach to training. Overemphasis on a single stroke or event can not only hinder overall growth but also increase the likelihood of physical and mental strain. By incorporating Curriculum-Based Training method that focuses on developing well-rounded young swimmers, coaches can help them reach their full potential while also safeguarding their physical and mental well-being.

Ultimately, the goal for coaches working with young swimmers should be to nurture their talent while prioritizing their long-term health and development. By distributing training time evenly across all competitive events, the Curriculum-Based Training method provides a balanced and sustainable training program for young swimmers. Emphasizing the importance of physical and technical diversity in training not only helps prevent overloading and injuries but also ensures that young swimmers stay engaged and motivated to continue improving in the sport.

Psychological Benefits and Motivation

The strategic distribution of training time among competitive events in swim training presents a range of psychological advantages for young swimmers. Embracing a Curriculum-Based Training season framework that emphasizes the equitable allotment of training time across all events enables young swimmers to derive a sense of achievement and advancement as they enhance their skills across different disciplines. This methodology cultivates a growth-oriented perspective, wherein young swimmers view each event as a chance for personal growth and skill refinement. Additionally, the balanced training regimen promotes discipline and dedication among swimmers, motivating them to consistently apply themselves across all facets of their training program.

Furthermore, the motivation of young swimmers is elevated by the strategic allocation of training time across all competitive events, fostering comprehensive skill development. By honing their proficiency in different strokes and distances, swimmers acquire a more profound insight into their strengths and areas for improvement. This heightened self-awareness not only fuels personal growth but also cultivates confidence and resilience to navigate obstacles effectively. The balanced skill set attained through equitable training time distribution enables young swimmers to confront each event with preparedness and flexibility, ultimately amplifying their overall performance and competitive advantage.

Ensuring a well-rounded distribution of training time across all competitive events is vital for safeguarding the psychological well-being of young swimmers in the long term. By Curriculum-Based Training season design and avoiding excessive focus on a single event, the risk of burnout or waning enthusiasm for the sport is minimized. This balanced approach not only mitigates physical strain but also fosters a positive mindset, enabling young swimmers to sustain a healthy perspective on their swimming endeavors. Embracing such a comprehensive training methodology supports a sustainable and gratifying athletic journey, buoying motivation and dedication among young swimmers as they progress in their competitive swimming pursuits.

BENEFITS OF IMPLEMENTING CURRICULUM-BASED TRAINING SEASON DESIGN

The Curriculum-Based Training approach presents a host of advantages for aspiring young swimmers seeking to excel in their competitive pursuits. Through the implementation of a meticulously planned swim season delineated into four-week intervals, focusing on key elements such as streamline, head/body alignment, breathing mechanics, and the pull phase, this method guarantees that young swimmers are afforded the opportunity to comprehensively delve into and refine their abilities. This methodical strategy equips young competitive swimmers with a profound comprehension of the technical intricacies of swimming, culminating in enhanced stroke mechanics and heightened water efficiency. Adherence to a structured season design empowers young swimmers to establish a robust groundwork for enduring success in competitive swimming, equipping them with the requisite proficiencies to excel across all facets of the sport.

CHAPTER 3
STRUCTURING EFFECTIVE SWIM PRACTICES

The key features of the Curriculum-Based Training program are as follows: The training method is specially tailored to mimic race day conditions by going over all of the tasks performed by the young swimmers. This approach emphasizes the establishment of solid competitive fundamentals in swimming, along with the cultivation of swimmers' self-correction abilities. Built on the principles of the spiral curriculum model, the structure of Curriculum-Based Training promotes efficient learning through its concentration on purposeful practice where prior skills attained are reviewed, recycled, and revised. A typical Curriculum-Based Training practice session is divided into three main components: Included in the structures are warm-up, training sets, and relays.

WARM-UP: ESTABLISHING DISCIPLINE AND FOCUS

The philosophy of warm-up in Curriculum-Based Training is based on Dr. Dave Salo's insights and underlines the significance of the effects of regular routines on athletes' performance. Therefore, sticking to the warm-up routine helps swimmers to develop routines, habits, and concentration. This is not just a warm-up; it is a way to train the mind to focus and get rid of any other thoughts that may interfere with practice sessions and competitions (Haugen & Seiler, 2019).

The structured warm-up routine assists young swimmers in cultivating a sense of readiness for both training and competitive swimming sessions. Participating in consistent warm-up procedures prior to each session helps to reinforce important values such as discipline and commitment. This repetition not only conditions their bodies for the physical task but also conditions their minds to be ready.

The warm-up routine involves repetitive sets that prove advantageous for swimmers by fostering concentration and readiness for the impending session. This enhances the swimmers' comfort and confidence, enabling them to approach training and competitions in a relaxed and focused state. Through consistent practice of the same warm-up routine, young swimmers are able to gain insights into their physical capacities and areas for improvement.

Therefore, the psychological advantages of a standardized warm-up go beyond the mere physical preparation of the body. It develops perseverance, focus, and determination, which are crucial virtues that are required in order to cope with the rigors of competitive swimming. In a team environment, the routine serves as more than just a warm-up; it is an integral component of the training culture that promotes team spirit, unity, and a shared goal among all team members.

Finally, it is the regularity of the warm-up regimen that creates the conditions for success in the pool. It provides a strong base from which a young swimmer can develop his or her skills, improve their efficiency, and achieve their best. By consistently sticking to a set routine, the coach and swimmers work together to efficiently foster a dedicated environment where progress through incremental improvements seamlessly integrates into the training regimen.

THE TRAINING SETS IN CURRICULUM-BASED TRAINING

In the realm of competitive swimming, success is often the culmination of systematic training, precise execution, and continuous improvement. The Curriculum-Based Training program stands as a testament to this approach, offering young swimmers a structured framework designed to elevate their competitive skills. At the core of the Curriculum-Based Training methodology lies the development of meticulously designed training sets rooted in the deliberate practice principles of Dr. Ericsson. These sets serve as essential building blocks in the cultivation of competitive skills. In view of swimming's competitive landscape and the necessity for productive training, it is recommended that each session incorporate three carefully planned training sets.

These sets are designed to correspond with the number of events that young swimmers race on average in a swim meet session. This deliberate structure not only prepares the young swimmer's body, but also prepares the mind to be able to handle the pressure of competition.

In Curriculum-Based Training, the organization of training sets is carefully crafted in alignment with the deliberate practice theory developed by Dr. Ericsson. This theory emphasizes methodical and concentrated practice for attaining expertise in a specific skill. Through the strategic arrangement of training sets, swimmers are guided in their pursuit of competitive skill mastery.

By employing a meticulously planned and targeted training set structure, young swimmers can seamlessly progress from basic to advanced competitive skills, leading to a consistent and substantial development. This well-organized approach not only fosters skill enhancement but also capitalizes on their current capabilities and experience. Through consistent improvement, young swimmers can elevate their competitive prowess and successfully reach their desired milestones.

Integrating Philosophy into Practice

Curriculum-Based Training emphasizes that deliberate practice equals effective practice because the focus is on acquiring and enhancing specific skills. The primary goals are to simulate real competitive scenarios and ensure the consistent improvement of young swimmers. By creating an environment that mirrors the challenges of actual competitions, swimmers can develop the physical and mental resilience required to excel under pressure.

A carefully designed practice session within the Curriculum-Based Training framework equips aspiring swimmers with essential skills for competitive swimming. This includes not only the technical aspects such as stroke efficiency and turn techniques but also the mental fortitude to handle the rigors of high-level competition. Additionally, the training instills valuable qualities like discipline, perseverance, and cooperation, which are integral to personal development. These attributes extend beyond the pool, helping swimmers become well-rounded individuals.

Coaches play a crucial role in this process, providing expert guidance to help swimmers embrace deliberate practice. They design training sessions that are challenging yet achievable, encouraging swimmers to push their limits while maintaining a focus on proper technical aspects. By offering constructive feedback and personalized coaching, they help each swimmer enhance their skill set and achieve optimal skill acquisition.

Moreover, the structured nature of Curriculum-Based Training ensures that practice is purposeful and goal-oriented. Each session is meticulously planned to target specific areas of improvement, fostering a sense of accomplishment and progress. This systematic approach not only improves performance but also builds confidence and a growth mindset in young swimmers.

By integrating these philosophies into daily practice, Curriculum-Based Training creates a nurturing and effective training environment. Young swimmers are encouraged to take ownership of their development, setting personal goals and working diligently to achieve them. This comprehensive approach ensures that young swimmers are well-prepared for the demands of competitive swimming and are equipped with the skills necessary for success both in and out of the water.

THE ROLE OF RELAYS IN CURRICULUM-BASED TRAINING

Swimming is a competitive sport: mastery doesn't consist of technical ability only; it requires the ability to work in teams, to strategize, and to build camaraderie. The last component of the Curriculum-Based Training method for young swimmers is the inclusion of relay races at the end of each practice session. It develops young swimmers who are versatile and who can perform well in both team and individual events.

Understanding the Philosophy Behind Relays

Relays in swimming are more than just an element of competition; they embody the synthesis of individual effort and collective success. In the Curriculum-Based Training framework, relays serve as a critical component for developing technical prowess and teamwork skills. The philosophy behind incorporating relays into Curriculum-Based Training is rooted in the understanding that mastering relay skills requires not only individual excellence but also seamless coordination and cooperation among team members.

To fully internalize relay skills, swimmers must practice them under conditions that closely mimic actual competitions.

Curriculum-Based Training recreates the environment of a swim meet, complete with the interactions, pressures, and dynamics of a race day. This simulation helps young swimmers acclimate to the stress and excitement of real competitions, ensuring they are mentally and physically prepared for the challenges they will face.

A core principle of Curriculum-Based Training is the repetition of skills to ensure mastery. Relays are strategically placed at the end of each practice session to test and reinforce the swimmers' technical abilities, as well as their understanding of team race tactics and strategies. This iterative approach allows young swimmers to build on their previous experiences, gradually refining their relay racing strategies. The repeated practice of dives, exchanges, and finishes within a relay context helps solidify these skills, making them second nature during actual competitions.

Relays require a high degree of coordination and synchronization among team members. Through regular practice, swimmers learn to trust and rely on one another, fostering a sense of unity and collective responsibility. This team-oriented practice helps young swimmers develop crucial interpersonal skills such as communication, cooperation, and mutual support. By working together towards a common goal, swimmers gain a deeper appreciation for the importance of teamwork and interdependence in achieving success.

Therefore, the races are designed not simply to enhance technical skills but also to instill a strategic mindset. Swimmers learn to make split-second decisions and adapt to the dynamic nature of relay races. They practice strategies such as optimal swimmer order, pacing, and efficient transitions. Understanding and executing these tactics are essential for maximizing team performance and gaining a competitive edge.

Practicing relays under simulated competition conditions helps build mental resilience. Swimmers learn to handle the pressure of performing in front of teammates and under the scrutiny of competition-like settings. This exposure helps reduce anxiety and build confidence, enabling young swimmers to maintain composure and focus during actual competition.

Benefits of Including Relays

1. Skill Enhancement and Mastery

> Relay races are a fundamental strategy for fostering self-reliance and teamwork skills among young swimmers. Each leg of the relay requires precise coordination, synchronization, and a basis of trust among team members. This systematic approach has proven to be highly effective in developing race-specific abilities.
>
> Participating in relay races offers young swimmers valuable developmental advantages, including enhanced reaction times and coordination skills. This advancement prepares them to competently engage in competition with increased efficiency, free from the constraints of excessive deliberation.

2. Teamwork and Camaraderie

> A significant component of Curriculum-Based Training rests on the principle of team building, predicated on the notion that young swimmers can greatly enhance their performance through peer support. Beyond its impact on individual achievements, relay races serve to foster unity and collaboration among team members. The essence of teamwork is cultivated through participation in relay events, providing a platform for mutual development and solidarity within the team.

Facilitating cooperation and enhancing comprehension among young swimmers is integral to fostering a collaborative environment. This approach transforms the process into a team-building exercise that imparts valuable life skills such as cooperation, leadership, and empathetic understanding. Undoubtedly, cultivating these attributes contributes greatly to the development and success of individuals within the swimming community.

3. Psychological Preparation

Relay events are valuable tools in the psychological preparation of swimmers for competition, offering them opportunities to simulate race scenarios. These races closely mirror the intensity of actual competition, effectively creating pressure and anticipation to better equip young swimmers for competitive environments. Coaches are advised to include relay races in training programs to teach crucial race strategies, develop effective pressure management skills, and enhance proficiency in race execution.

Implementation in Curriculum-Based Training

In Curriculum-Based Training, the relays are placed at the end of each practice session to recap the learning points and to also create a competition-like environment. It is crucial to understand that relay formats are chosen by coaches with great attention to the developmental needs of the swimmer and with a focus on the technical-tactical aspect of the race.

Besides, the introduction of relays also helps young swimmers improve their racing skill set while developing a competitive spirit based on cooperation. Coaches give feedback and suggestions to the swimmers after each relay, thereby enhancing the learning process of the young swimmer. We can see that the cyclical nature of skill acquisition and assessment is crucial in the formation of versatile swimmers capable of performing in solitary and group settings.

Building a Strong Foundation for Success

Integrating relays improves the coaches' capacity to cultivate racing skills and teamwork among young swimmers. Each relay session offers swimmers the chance to demonstrate their technical proficiency while working collaboratively.

In the realm of competitive swimming, the significance of teamwork cannot be overstated. By fostering a culture of cooperation and collaboration, swimmers are able to enhance their skills and achieve remarkable performance improvements. Through unwavering dedication and resilience, young swimmers not only improve their competitive edge but also cultivate strong interpersonal bonds that intertwine camaraderie with a spirit of healthy competition.

BENEFITS OF IMPLEMENTING CURRICULUM-BASED TRAINING FOR YOUNG SWIMMERS

Implementing the Curriculum-Based Training practice structure is a strategic method that enhances the growth of young swimmers by providing numerous benefits beyond physical conditioning. This system is crafted to mirror competitive racing dynamics and enhance the acquisition of advanced competitive skills. Emphasizing the systematic development of crucial skills, psychological robustness, and cohesive teamwork within a meticulously planned training schedule, this approach is designed to elevate overall skill development and foster excellence in young swimmers.

Replicating Race Day Conditions

As previously discussed, a fundamental aspect of Curriculum-Based Training involves replicating the competitive conditions and stresses faced by young swimmers during competitions. Structuring practices to mirror swim meets aids in preparing swimmers for the challenges inherent in a competitive environment. This approach not only facilitates the development of technical and racing proficiency but also provides valuable insight into the psychological and emotional demands of competitive swimming.

The practice structure in Curriculum-Based Training uses a spiral curriculum model that exposes the learner to a concept more than once, each time at a higher level. Every practice session is progressive in nature and enables the swimmers to gradually advance their knowledge of the stroke mechanics, racing strategies, and physical preparation. By integrating the spiral curriculum theory developed by Dr. Jerome S. Bruner with the concept of deliberate practice popularized by Dr. Anders Ericsson, Curriculum-Based Training aims to cultivate competency and confidence in young swimmers.

Comprehensive and Structured Training Regimen

Curriculum-Based Training organizes each practice session into distinct blocks: warm-up, training sets, and relays. This structured approach serves multiple purposes:

1. **Warm-Up**: The warm-up that has been recommended by the Curriculum-Based Training approach is not only a physical warm-up for the challenges that lie in front of the swimmers; it also creates a mental and emotional context for the focused training. Through the process of rituals in warm-up, young swimmers are made to have a routine and preparedness that leads to an improvement in their performance readiness.

2. **Training Sets:** In Curriculum-Based Training, the primary focuses revolve around skill development essential for a competitive environment. Each segment is specifically designed to advance throughout the season, gradually escalating the level of skill execution and difficulty. Swimmers are encouraged to push their limits, all the while improving fundamental skills. This deliberate practice methodology is remarkably adept at fostering incremental progress and ensuring that young swimmers are adequately prepared for the demands of training and competition.
3. **Relays**: The habit of having relay races after each practice is very significant as it brings out the aspects of teamwork and cooperation in swimming. Unlike the concept of individual events, relays involve swimmers working together, conveying information to one another, and having to make precise exchanges. Young swimmers learn relay racing strategies, as well as strengthening the team spirit that is so very essential in competitions.

Psychological and Social Benefits

In addition to developing technical skills, Curriculum-Based Training cultivates essential psychological attributes that are crucial in competitive swimming, as well as in personal development. The structured nature of Curriculum-Based Training greatly aids in fostering discipline, determination, and mental resilience among young swimmers. This framework enables swimmers to adhere to practice schedules, tackle challenges head-on, and cultivate a mindset of perseverance on their journey towards achievement.

The utilization of relays in Curriculum-Based Training enhances teamwork, communication, and camaraderie among participants. Relay activities require young swimmers to trust and depend on each other, fostering a culture of shared triumphs and setbacks that contribute to team development. This dynamic not only optimizes the training experience but also exposes young swimmers to competitive environments where collaboration is often the cornerstone of achievement.

Maximizing Potential and Achieving Goals

By embracing a Curriculum-Based Training practice structure, young swimmers are empowered to maximize their potential and achieve their goals in the pool. The systematic approach to skill development, coupled with a supportive coaching environment, enables young swimmers to progress steadily and confidently. Whether aiming for personal bests, qualifying for championships, or pursuing long-term athletic aspirations, Curriculum-Based Training equips swimmers with the tools and mindset needed to excel in the competitive world of swimming.

CHAPTER 4
TRAINING SET STRUCTURE

The training set design in Curriculum-Based Training utilizes three essential elements: deliberate practice for skill enhancement, a spiral curriculum model for holistic adaptation encompassing physiological and psychological aspects, and the blocked practice principle for proficiency in skill acquisition.

In Curriculum-Based Training, deliberate practice is a key component aimed at enhancing skills through focused and repetitive training sets. This method emphasizes the importance of breaking down complex skills into smaller, manageable tasks that are practiced consistently over time. By engaging in deliberate practice, young swimmers are able to rapidly improve on specific aspects of their performance, leading to a more efficient learning process and mastery of the desired skills. This approach allows for targeted and personalized training that caters to the young swimmers' unique needs, ultimately optimizing their development and progress in the training program.

Furthermore, the spiral curriculum model employed in Curriculum-Based Training facilitates a holistic approach to learning that encompasses not only physiological skills but also psychological aspects. This model acknowledges that learning is a continuous and interconnected process. With this in mind, the training sets are structured in a way that revisits and reinforces previous knowledge before progressing to more advanced concepts. By revisiting and building upon foundational skills in a systematic and strategic manner, young swimmers are able to develop a deep and comprehensive understanding of the skills performed. Additionally, by incorporating both physiological and psychological elements into the training sets, swimmers are better equipped to cope with the various challenges and demands they may encounter during their training journey.

In addition, the blocked practice principle plays a crucial role in training sets by promoting proficiency in skill acquisition. This principle involves grouping similar tasks together and dedicating focused training sets to a specific skill. By organizing training in this manner, young swimmers are able to concentrate on mastering one skill at a time, which leads to more efficient and effective skill acquisition. The blocked practice principle enables young swimmers to develop a strong foundation in each skill before moving on to more complex or challenging tasks, which ultimately enhances their competency in the training.

Anders Ericsson's Deliberate Practice Principles

Curriculum-Based Training focuses on constructing training sets with a strong emphasis on deliberate practice. This approach fosters a structured and systematic way of developing skills. By deconstructing complex skills into manageable tasks, young swimmers can concentrate on refining specific aspects of the skill required for their advancement.

To achieve ongoing progress in each training set, young swimmers focus on refining crucial technical stroke elements and specific event requirements such as turns, breathing patterns, and determining optimal effort levels. Purposeful practice of these fundamentals over time allows young swimmers to elevate their overall stroke proficiency and competitive skills required for all events.

Training sets in Curriculum-Based Training reduce the time required to develop stroke mechanics and racing proficiency across all events. This results in heightened water efficiency that parallels overall performance improvements.

Deliberate practice is essential in training sets as it allows young swimmers to excel in areas that need improvement and to dedicate focused time and effort to mastering those skills. Dr. Ericsson believes this intentional and repetitive training approach helps create more gray matter for a specific skill and increases proficiency, enabling young swimmers to race effectively during competitions. By tailoring training sets to align with the specific needs of each racing event, young swimmers will develop a deep understanding of the demands and requirements of their races, leading to increased confidence and strategic race execution.

Moreover, the personalized nature of deliberate practice in the training sets ensures that young swimmers receive targeted instruction and feedback tailored to their individual strengths and weaknesses. This individualized approach not only optimizes skill development but also nurtures a sense of ownership and accountability in young swimmers with regard to their progress and growth. By instilling a culture of discipline and focused practice, remarkable results can be achieved. Training sets that are designed in accordance with Curriculum-Based Training will cultivate a strong work ethic and a commitment to continuous improvement. This leads to a solid foundation for success both in and out of the water.

How the Spiral Curriculum Model Fits in

The spiral curriculum model is a dynamic approach that recognizes the importance of revisiting and reinforcing fundamental skills before moving on to more advanced concepts. The cyclical progression of the training sets within the Curriculum-Based Training method allows young swimmers to develop a strong foundation and gradually build upon their knowledge and abilities over time. By revisiting the same training sets at regular intervals, swimmers are able to deepen their understanding and mastery of skills, enhancing their overall learning experience. This intentional repetition not only reinforces technical skills but also instills confidence and resilience in young swimmers as they navigate the complexities of training.

Moreover, the holistic nature of the training sets integrates both physiological and psychological elements, enriching the learning journey for young swimmers. By addressing not only the physical aspects of swimming skills but also the mental components such as focus, confidence, and resilience, swimmers are equipped with a wide and comprehensive skill set. This integrated approach enhances the effectiveness of training and prepares swimmers to cope with the mental challenges and pressures that inevitably arise during competitions or intensive training sessions. By fostering incremental skill development, the spiral curriculum model-inspired training sets in the Curriculum-Based Training system ensure that young swimmers are well-rounded with the tools to excel in any environment.

In addition, the systematic and strategic approach within the training set design promotes a deeper and more meaningful understanding of competitive swimming skills among young swimmers. By breaking down complex technical skills into manageable components and gradually building upon them, swimmers are supported in their skill acquisition and progression. The structured approach of the training sets not only enhances skill retention and application but also fosters a sense of accomplishment and motivation as the swimmers see tangible progress in their performance. As a result, the

Curriculum-Based Training sets ensure that young swimmers develop a solid technical foundation, a resilient mindset, and, very likely, a love for the sport that will last a lifetime.

Blocked Training

The utilization of the blocked practice principle is highly advantageous for young swimmers, as it facilitates the gradual enhancement of their skills and boosts their confidence. By deconstructing training sessions into smaller, focused tasks, swimmers can effectively monitor and appreciate their progress, thus fostering continuous improvement.

The feeling of achievement enhances their motivation and solidifies the learning process. Focusing on a single skill at a time in accordance with the blocked practice principle helps young swimmers develop a thorough understanding of the fundamental and technical elements. This approach fosters a robust foundation for their skill development. Establishing a strong foundation is paramount for the acquisition of advanced skills in the future.

The blocked practice principle enhances the retention of skills and knowledge. By repeatedly practicing the same skill in a concentrated manner, swimmers are more likely to create and retain neural connections necessary for executing the skill correctly. This repetitive practice reinforces the connections in the brain related to that specific skill, making it easier for swimmers to recall and perform the skill accurately in future training sessions and competitions. This retention of skills is crucial for building a consistent swimmer in the long term, ensuring that young swimmers can continue to progress and grow in their swimming abilities.

Furthermore, the blocked practice principle helps young swimmers develop a systematic approach to their training sets, allowing them to effectively manage their time and effort during practice sessions. By focusing on one skill at a time, swimmers can set clear goals and benchmarks for mastering each skill before moving on to the next task. This structured approach not only improves their overall skill development but also instills a sense of discipline and dedication in young swimmers. Learning to prioritize and allocate time for focused practice under the blocked practice principle teaches valuable time management skills that can be applied not only in swimming but also in other aspects of their lives.

SUMMARY AND COACHES' BENEFITS OF CURRICULUM-BASED TRAINING SETS

Swim coaches can experience sizable gains by utilizing Curriculum-Based Training in the form of deliberate practice, the spiral curriculum model, and the blocked practice principle when structuring training sets for young swimmers. The aforementioned methods collectively contribute to the development of skills, and the refinement of execution of training, thus making the training sessions more effective.

Deliberate Practice

By integrating deliberate practice into training set design, coaches can optimize skill development for young swimmers through a systematic and focused approach. Deliberate practice is characterized by its targeted nature, where each training session is meticulously planned to address specific performance components. This strategy is particularly effective for rapidly improving distinct skills and mechanics, elements that are essential for competitive swimming.

Tailored deliberate practice is a specialized training approach designed to meet the unique needs of every young swimmer. Coaches analyze the strengths and weaknesses of each individual swimmer to design training sets that target and improve specific areas of their performance.

The personalized focus offered to each swimmer enables them to make progress and enhance their skills by receiving tailored training. Coaches give consistent feedback to help swimmers improve their mechanics and make any required modifications. This ongoing cycle of practice, feedback, and correction is central to deliberate practice. It results in a steady fostering of consistent growth.

Coaches support young swimmers in making remarkable advancements across all areas of competitive swimming by focusing on fundamental skills through intentional and consistent practice. These improvements encompass not only technical elements like stroke mechanics and turns but also strategic components like race pacing and mental resilience.

Spiral Curriculum Model

Implementing the concept of a spiral curriculum is beneficial for young swimmers as it implies that every new concept is accompanied by the repeated practice of previous training sessions. In this context, young swimmers are encouraged to thoroughly analyze all aspects of competitive swimming and ensure that their physical comprehension is complemented by a strong mental understanding. Regular review of training sets enables young swimmers to cultivate fundamental skills essential for success in advanced training sessions and competitive environments.

Spiral curriculum is progressive in nature, which means that young swimmers' knowledge and skills are increased gradually and their confidence and perseverance are enhanced. Utilizing this model ensures that coaches provide training in a variety of fundamental skills, preparing swimmers to adapt to diverse swimming conditions effectively.

Blocked Practice Principle

The application of the blocked practice principle is fundamental in Curriculum-Based Training sets as it significantly improves the efficacy of skill acquisition in young swimmers. This principle mandates that during training sessions, young swimmers concentrate on mastering one skill at a time. By compartmentalizing similar tasks, coaches can ensure that swimmers attain proficiency before progressing to more intricate skills.

Establishing a consistent and structured swim training regimen is imperative for young competitive swimmers. The blocked practice method in training set design has shown itself to be effective in improving skill retention and motivation. Implementing blocked practice set design enables coaches to assist swimmers in building confidence, promoting consistency, and effectively tracking progress in mastering essential swimming skills.

Practical Implementation

Systematic planning of Curriculum-Based Training sets ensures that young swimmers receive tailored and effective training that addresses their individual needs and goals. By conducting a detailed evaluation of each swimmer's skill level and potential for development, coaches can identify areas for improvement and create targeted training sets to help young swimmers reach their full potential. This personalized approach not only maximizes the effectiveness of training sessions but also keeps swimmers motivated and engaged in their training.

Active participation from coaches is essential in implementing Curriculum-Based Training sets successfully. Coaches play a critical role in guiding young swimmers through their training, providing feedback, and monitoring progress toward set goals. Also, by engaging in the planning and execution of training sets, coaches demonstrate their commitment to the development of their swimmers and can make real-time adjustments to ensure that training sessions are challenging yet achievable. This collaborative approach between coaches and swimmers fosters a supportive training environment that promotes growth, skill development, and success in competitive swimming.

CHAPTER 5
A COMPREHENSIVE APPROACH TO SKILL DEVELOPMENT IN CURRICULUM-BASED TRAINING

The Curriculum-Based Training approach incorporates a unique single drill system for stroke development, setting it apart from traditional training methodologies. Drawing inspiration from Dr. Jerome S. Bruner's spiral curriculum model and Dr. Anders Ericsson's deliberate practice, this approach is designed to optimize the learning experience and skill enhancement of young swimmers. Emphasizing critical elements such as streamline, head and body position, breathing mechanics, and pull phase, this methodology provides swimmers with a structured framework for mastering each aspect of their strokes. By fostering a deep understanding and proficiency in these fundamentals, swimmers are guided towards a more efficient pathway to skill mastery.

Utilizing well-established scientific principles, the Curriculum-Based Training approach strategically harmonizes learning methodologies with the developmental requirements of young swimmers. Through a focused emphasis on key aspects of stroke refinement via the single drill system, young swimmers can systematically and intensively augment their skill set. This approach not only cultivates enhanced technical proficiency among young swimmers but also lays a robust groundwork for future progress and advancement in their swimming capabilities.

The single drill system presents a streamlined and effective approach to enhancing swimming skills. By carefully selecting the suitable drill and establishing a specific number of blocks that it will be applied to, swimmers are able to concentrate on individual elements of their strokes to optimize their skill acquisition. This methodical strategy offers young swimmers a well-organized and rigorous training routine, fostering the development and mastery of their abilities. Through a dedicated focus on stroke development and consistency, the single drill system offers a pragmatic and successful trajectory for progress.

Philosophical Foundations of the Single Drill System

The single drill system is a fundamental component of the Curriculum-Based Training program, founded upon the principles of deliberate practice as espoused by renowned psychologist Dr. Anders Ericsson. This approach emphasizes the importance of focused and intentional practice for attaining high levels of proficiency. It underscores the necessity for training to be purposeful and targeted rather than just a simple repetition. By prioritizing precision and dedicating substantial time to refining specific skill sets, this method empowers young swimmers to enhance their abilities progressively.

Emphasizing Deliberate Practice

Deliberate practice is a highly effective and focused method aimed at markedly improving specific skills. It means young swimmers are engaged in tailored drills to enhance foundational skills. By concentrating on aspects such as head position or breathing mechanics within a single drill, young swimmers can effectively elevate their stroke mechanics. With precise guidance from coaches, swimmers can refine their strokes without the confusion of juggling multiple drills. This approach facilitates quicker and more substantial improvements in stroke development.

The framework of deliberate practice entails the strategic provision of targeted feedback to young swimmers throughout their training sessions. Coaches play an essential role in attentively observing and delivering constructive feedback, facilitating young swimmers' understanding and skill development. This feedback loop fosters a culture of continuous learning and progress. The focus is on achieving mastery of distinctive skills within each drill before progressing further, ensuring a high degree of proficiency. This approach serves as the cornerstone for subsequent skill refinement and enhancement.

Integrating the Principle of Specificity

The single drill system is built on the concept of specificity and deliberate practice. This principle emphasizes that practice must mirror the performance objectives as closely as possible. Essentially, each drill within the single drill system is designed to closely replicate the desired performance. Competitive strokes are undertaken with a specific and efficient approach. This method focuses on developing skills during drill practice sessions that are essential for competitive situations.

The principle of specificity, when applied within the single drill system, significantly improves young swimmers' efficiency in all aspects of their stroke. By engaging in targeted training that focuses on specific mechanical elements, swimmers can deepen their understanding of their stroke and develop the necessary neural pathways in the brain. This strategic and focused approach allows swimmers to master essential skills, which leads to increased efficiency in the pool. Ultimately, this method contributes to comprehensive improvement in all facets of the sport.

Structured Framework for Skill Enhancement

Thus, by incorporating Dr. Ericsson's deliberate practice principle with the specificity principle, the single drill system provides a strong and systematic approach to achieving a competitive skill set. It ensures that young swimmers undergo well-directed and well-intended practice sessions in relation to their performance intentions. The single drill system is systematic, and swimmers are able to build their skills and confidence gradually.

The drills in the single drill system are meticulously selected to meet the specific needs of aspiring competitive swimmers. Each drill for every stroke is tailored to match the developmental capacities of young athletes, ensuring practice sessions are purposeful and productive. This targeted approach minimizes the risk of wasted time and effort, facilitating continuous improvement and skill development.

Impact on Mindset and Approach

The philosophical foundations of the single drill system also influence the mindset and approach that young swimmers adopt during training. By emphasizing the importance of deliberate and specific practice, swimmers learn to approach their training with a sense of purpose and discipline. They understand that each drill is an opportunity to refine their skills and make tangible progress toward their goals.

This mindset fosters a culture of continuous improvement and resilience. Young swimmers are encouraged to embrace challenges and view them as opportunities for growth. The focused nature of the single drill system helps swimmers develop a strong work ethic and a commitment to excellence, both of which are essential for achieving success in competitive swimming.

IMPLEMENTATION IN CURRICULUM-BASED TRAINING

Principle of Specificity

Integrating a single drill system into the Curriculum-Based Training is a strategic decision that emphasizes the importance of specificity in skill development. The principle of specificity is a foundational concept in sports training, emphasizing the need to align training drills with the required skills and objectives. The principle of specificity is essential, as it recognizes the individualized adaptation of the body to stress. Therefore, it's imperative to tailor training drills to closely replicate the desired skill or technical element. This approach is particularly valuable when incorporated into the training regimen of young swimmers.

By participating in the single drill system that replicates the precise movements necessary for competitive strokes, young swimmers can enhance their stroke mechanics with higher skill retainment. It allows them to make fine adjustments to many facets of the stroke, such as body position or timing of the stroke. It has been established that when these skills are taken through practice sessions and then into competitive races, the emphasis on consistent and focused training enhances the performance of swimmers.

Deliberate Practice Principle

Deliberate practice is characterized by dedicating attention to specific tasks and consistently challenging young swimmers to enhance their proficiency. In the Curriculum-Based Training method, adhering to a singular drill over an extended duration, such as two training blocks or longer, forms a cornerstone for developing competitive strokes. This prolonged commitment enables young swimmers to fully engage with the nuances of the drill, thereby sharpening their abilities and perfecting their stroke efficiency.

Through consistent practice of repetitive drills, young swimmers not only gain familiarity with the targeted drills but also cultivate the ability to make adjustments and self-correct their form. This process of internalizing the correct stroke mechanics is essential for solidifying the movements as inherent skills.

Furthermore, it ensures that skills learned during training sessions are transferred to competitions after some time of practice. The young swimmers who devote plenty of time to practicing these drills are in a better position to handle themselves during competitions.

Consequently, the deliberate practice concept of repeating a particular drill for an extensive amount of time sharpens the skills of young swimmers and builds a strong base of proper stroke mechanics. This methodical single drill system sustains progressive development and ensures younger swimmers are prepared for a competitive environment.

Spiral Curriculum Model

Applying Dr. Jerome S. Bruner's spiral curriculum into the strokes' development for young swimmers is another effective way of providing a progressive way of improving fundamental skills. As young swimmers progress through different training blocks, they are introduced to increasingly challenging levels of stroke fundamentals. This method fosters a continuous learning process whereby young swimmers cyclically engage with and expand upon mastered competencies, resulting in a spiral effect of skill development.

The application of the spiral curriculum principle in the progression of skills in stroke development ensures there is continuity and ease as the young swimmers transfer from one level of development to another. By applying this method, it's possible to gain a complete understanding of the constituent parts of each stroke, which strengthens the general foundation that underpins effective swimming.

In this manner, through a single-drill system planned in such a way that a particular set of drills is conducted during the competitive season, young swimmers are systematically improving their abilities. They achieve long-term and holistic improvements in their stroke development. The essence of foundational skills becomes challenging in the subsequent blocks, which creates the 'spiral effect,' allowing young swimmers to develop the acquired competencies further and progress to mastering advanced stroke elements. It also enables a gradual build-up from the simple aspects of stroke skills to the complex, making sure that a comprehensive and permanent improvement in the general structure of the stroke is achieved.

By utilizing the single drill system, the Curriculum-Based Training method integrates the spiral curriculum model to optimize stroke development for young swimmers. This approach of constructing strong fundamentals for young swimmers provides for constant progress and achievements in their swimming careers.

BUILDING MASTERY THROUGH STROKE DEVELOPMENT

Curriculum-Based Training employs a single and specific drill method for stroke improvement while eliminating multiple-drill swimming training methods. This methodology provides a focused and detailed method of skill enhancement. Unlike the usual training that includes various types of drills, the Curriculum-Based Training minimizes learning factors that slow down the development of skills. It allows young swimmers to systematically focus on individual components of their strokes, facilitating a deeper understanding and improved stroke mechanics over time. Traditional multiple-drill training procedures have a tendency to spread concentration in different directions, reducing the factors of depth and accuracy that are crucial for development.

Integrating Scientific Principles

The Curriculum-Based Training method is based on the scientific findings of experts like Dr. Jerome S. Bruner and Dr. Anders Ericsson. It's characterized by its spiral curriculum model and deliberate practice, which are incorporated into the single drill system. The spiral curriculum model provides cyclic coverage, ensuring that young swimmers are introduced to fundamental concepts at varying levels of complexity. This methodology enables them to develop a strong foundation in competitive swimming by progressively building upon their knowledge and skills.

Deliberate practice, according to Dr. Ericsson, consists of intensive and continuous training accompanied by feedback. This, he believes, is essential for enhancing complex skills. The single drill system is appropriate to the development of strokes and is distinguished from random pattern training. In contrast to broad multi-drill swimming approaches, Curriculum-Based Training fosters a higher level of precision in skill acquisition.

Advantages of a Single Drill System

The incorporation of the single drill system in Curriculum-Based Training signifies a significant advancement in swimming instruction, emphasizing the precision and effectiveness of training drills. By meticulously targeting the specific movements essential for each stroke, young swimmers are able to cultivate a profound comprehension allied to high levels of muscle memory with regard to correct form. This approach elevates the proficiency of young swimmers and mitigates the potential for injuries stemming from improper stroke mechanics or excessive training.

By customizing drills to closely simulate the precise movements essential for competitive swimming strokes, young swimmers can enhance their ability to internalize and execute correct stroke mechanics during competition. This focused strategy not only enhances stroke mechanics but also fosters greater skill retention over time.

The structured approach of the single drill system highlights the significance of precision and consistency in training. This method avoids inundating young swimmers with numerous drills that may not align with their specific requirements, instead facilitating a targeted and intentional strategy for enhancing skills. Through dedicated practice of specific motor movements, young swimmers can significantly improve their stroke mechanics and make substantial advancements in their training.

CHAPTER 6
PSYCHOLOGY AND COMPETITION

A common challenge faced by young swimmers in competitive environments is performance anxiety. The pressure of meeting personal and external expectations, combined with the competitive nature of the sport, can lead to increased levels of stress and anxiety. This might manifest in symptoms such as nervousness, self-doubt, and a fear of underperformance and can significantly impact the athlete's overall performance. The Curriculum-Based Training approach aims to provide strategies for effectively managing these emotions, improving focus, and fostering optimal performance. The development of a resilient mindset is imperative for young swimmers to effectively overcome this obstacle.

A prevalent psychological challenge faced by young swimmers during competitions is the tendency to compare themselves with their peers. It's typical of swimmers to evaluate themselves against others with regard to speed, stroke efficiency, and accomplishments. This comparison has the potential to evoke emotions such as insecurity, inadequacy, or jealousy, which may divert their attention from their individual performance and objectives. The Curriculum-Based Training method assists young swimmers in redirecting their attention from external comparisons and toward internal progression and personal development. In this way, it bolsters their mental fortitude and self-assurance, and encourages confidence in their own skills and performance level.

Ensuring the perpetuation of motivation and fortitude can be psychologically difficult for young swimmers. The rigorous physical exertion inherent to competitive swimming, coupled with the relentless mental stresses of the contest, are often strenuous and fatiguing. Maintaining motivation, concentration, and perseverance becomes a formidable task, particularly in the face of adversity or impediments encountered during races. The Curriculum-Based Training method cultivates mental tactics, establishing achievable objectives, and nurturing a resilient mindset. These are essential components that enable young swimmers to surmount the hurdles and excel optimally in competitive environments.

Overall, the use of the psychology of words and triggers in the Curriculum-Based Training method helps young swimmers develop a positive mindset, manage competition-induced anxiety, and improve their overall performance in competitive settings. By creating a supportive and empowering training environment, coaches can help young swimmers build the mental skills necessary to excel in competitions and achieve their full potential.

REDUCING ANXIETY

Curriculum-Based Training, based on spiral curriculum and deliberate practice, plays a crucial role in helping young swimmers cope with anxiety during competitions by reducing unknown factors. The spiral curriculum approach involves revisiting and building upon previously learned skills, allowing swimmers to gradually master and internalize them over time. This iterative process helps in instilling confidence and reducing uncertainty, which are common triggers for anxiety in competitive situations.

Furthermore, deliberate practice involves breaking down complex skills into smaller elements and repetitively practicing them with focused attention and feedback. By engaging in deliberate practice, young swimmers can enhance their self-efficacy and competence, leading to a sense of control over their performance. This structured approach not only improves technical proficiency but also cultivates mental resilience, enabling swimmers to better deal with the pressures of competition.

Additionally, the Curriculum-Based Training program offers young swimmers a complete range of resources and strategies to effectively handle anxiety and foster positive self-talk. By integrating these tools into their training routines, swimmers acquire the ability to control their emotions, exhibit composure, and concentrate on their performance objectives while navigating through the unpredictable environment of competition. This proactive methodology empowers young swimmers with the essential competencies required to cope with unfamiliar or demanding situations, thereby mitigating the potential influence of unforeseen variables on their performance outcomes.

Overall, by combining the principles of spiral curriculum and deliberate practice, the Curriculum-Based Training offers a holistic framework for young swimmers to build their mental and physical capacities, ultimately enhancing their ability to cope with anxiety and perform at their best in competitive environments.

PEER PRESSURE

Curriculum-Based Training, particularly when rooted in the principles of spiral curriculum and deliberate practice, plays a pivotal role in helping young swimmers manage the psychological challenges associated with unfavorable comparisons during competitive events. By addressing both the technical and mental aspects of training, the Curriculum-Based Training method equips swimmers with the skills and mindset necessary to navigate the pressures of competition in a healthy and constructive manner.

The spiral curriculum framework is designed to introduce and revisit fundamental skills and principles in a systematic and iterative fashion. This method ensures that swimmers build a solid foundation of knowledge and competencies that are reinforced and expanded upon. Each iteration allows swimmers to deepen their understanding and refine their competitive skills, which not only enhances their technical proficiency but also promotes a mindset of continuous improvement. This progressive approach helps swimmers internalize the idea that mastery is a gradual process, thereby reducing the pressure to achieve immediate perfection and mitigating the anxiety associated with peer comparisons.

Deliberate practice, a core component of Curriculum-Based Training, involves targeted and purposeful training that focuses on addressing individual weaknesses while enhancing strengths. This approach encourages young swimmers to set attainable goals, identify areas for improvement, and work diligently to advance their skills. By emphasizing personal development and growth, deliberate practice shifts the focus away from external benchmarks and toward individual progress. This fosters a growth-oriented mindset, where swimmers learn to value their efforts and improvements instead of measuring their success against their peers.

Engaging in deliberate practice enables swimmers to establish a personal baseline and track their development. This process helps them recognize their unique progress and celebrate their achievements, no matter how small. By concentrating on their own journey, swimmers are less likely to feel insecure, inadequate, or jealous when comparing themselves to others. Instead, they develop a sense of pride in their individual accomplishments and a more resilient attitude towards competition.

Curriculum-Based Training also incorporates a range of psychological tools and strategies to help young swimmers manage the emotional challenges associated with peer pressure. One key aspect is the emphasis on internal progression and personal milestones. By focusing on their own growth and achievements, swimmers learn to appreciate their unique strengths and capabilities. This shift in perspective fosters a healthier approach to competition, where the emphasis is on self-improvement rather than outperforming others.

Additionally, Curriculum-Based Training includes techniques for fostering positive self-talk and emotional regulation. Swimmers are taught to recognize and challenge negative thoughts that stem from unfavorable comparisons. By developing skills in mindfulness and emotional control, they can maintain composure and focus during competitions, reducing the impact of peer pressure on their performance.

The combination of the spiral curriculum and deliberate practice within the Curriculum-Based Training method not only improves technical skills but also builds mental fortitude and self-assurance. Young swimmers learn to view competition as an opportunity to become stronger and better rather than a measure of how others see their worth. This mindset empowers them to handle the pressures of competition with greater confidence and resilience.

By reinforcing the value of personal growth and internal progression, Curriculum-Based Training helps young swimmers develop a potent sense of self-worth that isn't dependent on external validation. This intrinsic motivation is crucial for sustaining long-term engagement and enjoyment in the sport. Swimmers who are confident in their abilities and committed to their personal development are more likely to persevere through challenges and setbacks, ultimately achieving higher levels of performance. So, this approach of encouraging self-worth often does, in fact, lead to excellent results in competitions.

MAINTAINING MOTIVATION

Curriculum-Based Training, based on spiral curriculum and deliberate practice, as well as the principle of specificity, plays a crucial role in helping young swimmers develop motivation for competitions. The spiral curriculum approach emphasizes continuous revisiting and building upon fundamental skills, which helps swimmers gradually improve and master their abilities. By consistently reviewing and reinforcing essential swimming concepts, young swimmers are better equipped to tackle the challenges of competition with confidence.

Deliberate practice within the Curriculum-Based Training ensures that swimmers engage in purposeful and focused training sessions that target specific areas for improvement. Through deliberate practice, swimmers can refine their strokes, develop a competitive skill set, and sharpen their mental acuity, all of which are essential for success in competitive swimming. This systematic approach to training allows young swimmers to track their progress, set achievable goals, and see tangible improvements over time, which in turn boosts their motivation and drive to excel in competitions.

Moreover, the principle of specificity within Curriculum-Based Training tailors training programs to mimic the demands of actual competitive events. By structuring training sessions to replicate race conditions, young swimmers can familiarize themselves with the physical and mental challenges they will face when competing. This specificity helps swimmers develop the necessary skills, strategies, and mindset required during competition.

By combining the principles of spiral curriculum, deliberate practice, and specificity, the Curriculum-Based Training system provides young swimmers with a comprehensive and effective framework for skill development and competition preparation. Through this structured and holistic approach, young swimmers can cultivate the motivation, resilience, and determination needed to thrive in the competitive swimming arena.

POWER OF WORDS

Words have a unique ability to shape our thoughts and emotions. In competitive settings, such as swimming, the language used by coaches, parents, and even the athletes themselves, can significantly affect psychological states. Positive and empowering words enhance confidence and focus, while negative or critical language exacerbates anxiety, insecurity, and self-doubt. Recognizing this, Curriculum-Based Training leverages the psychology of words to foster a more resilient and optimistic mindset in young swimmers.

Positive reinforcement involves affirming desired behaviors and attitudes through encouraging language and actions. In the context of Curriculum-Based Training, this means consistently using words that highlight a swimmer's strengths and improvements instead of their shortcomings. For example, instead of saying, "Don't be slow off the blocks," a coach might say, "Quick and powerful off the blocks!" This shift in phrasing helps swimmers focus on positive actions and outcomes, reducing anxiety associated with potential failures.

Trigger words are carefully selected terms designed to evoke specific emotional and physiological responses that enhance performance. These words are integrated into training routines and competitions to help swimmers maintain focus, boost confidence, and manage stress. Words like "strong," "focused," and "resilient" are commonly used to instill a sense of capability and determination. When these words are repeated consistently, they become internalized, triggering automatic positive responses in high-pressure situations.

A resilient mindset is crucial for young swimmers to navigate the pressures of competition. By incorporating empowering language into daily training, the Curriculum-Based Training method helps swimmers develop mental toughness. Coaches might use phrases like "You are prepared," "Trust your training," to reinforce the swimmer's belief in their abilities. Over time, these affirmations can significantly bolster a swimmer's self-confidence and reduce anxiety.

Practical Applications in Training and Competition

- **Daily Practice Sessions**: During regular training sessions, coaches can incorporate trigger words and positive reinforcement in feedback and instructions. Phrases like "excellent progress," "keep pushing," and "look at that improvement" create a positive learning environment where swimmers feel supported and motivated.
- **Pre-Competition Routines**: Before competitions, coaches can help swimmers develop personalized mantras or affirmations that include their trigger words. This practice helps swimmers enter the competition with a positive and focused mindset, reducing pre-race anxiety.
- **In-Competition Strategies**: During competitions, quick verbal cues from coaches using trigger words can help swimmers stay focused and calm. Simple affirmations like "strong finish" or "stay focused" can make a significant difference in maintaining composure under pressure.
- **Post-Competition Reflection**: After competitions, using positive language to review performances helps young swimmers focus on their successes and areas for

improvement without feeling criticized. Constructive feedback, framed positively, encourages ongoing development and resilience.

The strategic use of positive language extends beyond individual performance. It fosters a team culture where encouragement and support are the norms. When swimmers hear positive and empowering words from their coaches and teammates, it creates a collective environment of mutual respect and motivation. This culture not only enhances individual performances, it also strengthens team cohesion and morale.

PSYCHOLOGY OF WORDS IN CURRICULUM-BASED TRAINING

The science behind the psychology of words acknowledges the intricate ways in which language can impact our cognitive processes, emotions, and behavior. In the context of the Curriculum-Based Training method for young swimmers, the use of specific trigger words is grounded in psychological principles aimed at reducing competition-induced anxiety and enhancing performance.

Words have the power to evoke strong emotional responses and can influence the way young swimmers perceive and interpret situations. In competitive settings like swimming, where pressure and stress are common, the choice of words used by coaches can significantly impact the athletes' mental state. Positive and empowering words instill confidence, boost motivation, and foster a sense of resilience in young swimmers, helping them navigate the challenges of competition with a more constructive mindset.

Through the process of positive reinforcement, which involves rewarding desired behaviors with praise or encouragement, the Curriculum-Based Training method leverages the psychology of words to create a supportive and nurturing environment. By consistently reinforcing positive associations with specific words or phrases, coaches can help shape young swimmers' thought patterns and emotional responses, leading to improved performance and overall well-being.

Furthermore, the psychology of words also highlights the importance of self-talk and internal dialog in shaping swimmers's beliefs and attitudes. By encouraging young swimmers to adopt positive self-affirmations and internalize empowering language, the method aims to cultivate a mindset of self-efficacy and resilience, enabling athletes to overcome challenges and setbacks with greater determination and composure.

In essence, the integration of psychology and language in the Curriculum-Based Training method underscores the profound impact words have on a young swimmer's psychology and performance. By harnessing the science of words to promote positivity, confidence, and mental strength, coaches will help young swimmers unlock their full potential and thrive in competitive environments.

LONG-TERM BENEFITS

The long-term benefits of implementing Curriculum-Based Training to address performance anxiety and psychological challenges during competitions are numerous and significant. Here are some of the key long-term benefits:

Increased Mental Resilience: By providing strategies for managing emotions and developing a resilient mindset, Curriculum-Based Training equips young swimmers with the mental strength to cope with anxiety not only in competitions but also in various aspects of their lives. Over time, this resilience can enhance their ability to face challenges and bounce back from setbacks effectively.

Improved Focus and Concentration: The training approach helps young swimmers improve their focus and concentration by redirecting their attention from external comparisons to internal progression and personal development. This enhanced focus can benefit them not only in swimming competitions but also in academics and other areas requiring concentrated effort.

Sustained Motivation and Perseverance: By cultivating mental tactics and setting achievable objectives, Curriculum-Based Training supports young swimmers in staying motivated and persevering through the adversities encountered during races. These qualities of motivation and perseverance will translate into long-term success and achievement in swimming and other endeavors.

Enhanced Self-Efficacy and Confidence: Through deliberate practice and the reinforcement of positive self-talk, young swimmers will enhance their self-efficacy and competence. Over time, this enhanced confidence can permeate all aspects of their lives, leading to greater self-assurance and belief in their abilities to overcome challenges.

Development of Growth Mindset: The approach of the Curriculum-Based Training method encourages a growth-oriented mindset focused on personal development rather than external benchmarks. This mindset shift fosters a continuous desire for improvement, learning, and progress, which can benefit young swimmers in their athletic pursuits and in their personal and professional growth.

Improved Coping Skills and Stress Management: By providing tools to effectively handle anxiety and stress, Curriculum-Based Training equips young swimmers with valuable coping skills that will serve them far beyond their swimming careers. Learning to manage stress in high-pressure situations leads to better emotional regulation and mental well-being in many life situations.

Long-Term Performance Enhancement: Through the structured and holistic approach of the Curriculum-Based Training, young swimmers can continuously improve their skills and mental resilience. This long-term focus on skill development can lead to sustained performance enhancement, ultimately helping them achieve their full potential in competitive swimming and other pursuits.

In summary, the implementation of Curriculum-Based Training methods will produce enduring benefits in young swimmers that extend well beyond their time in the pool. By nurturing essential psychological skills, fostering positive mindset shifts, and instilling a growth-oriented approach to challenges, this training method can play a pivotal role in shaping the overall well-being and success of young swimmers in the long term.

CONCLUSION

The Comprehensive Curriculum-Based Training for Young Competitive Swimmers presents a cutting-edge methodology that regards swimmers as lifelong learners on a journey of advancement and maturation. Drawing upon insights from esteemed theorists such as Dr. Jerome S. Bruner and Dr. Anders Ericsson, this approach emphasizes gradual advancement and enhancement in the pursuit of flawlessness.

Through the Curriculum-Based Training method, a fresh coaching perspective for young swimmers is introduced, integrating progressive skills and mental preparation based on the principles of ongoing learning and skill acquisition. With a comprehensive focus on physical, cognitive, and psychological dimensions, this strategy equips young swimmers for a fun and challenging journey in competitive swimming while cultivating a growth-oriented outlook and a dedication to continual progress. By promoting self-awareness, structured training, and purposeful practice, coaches empower young swimmers to realize their utmost potential both in the aquatic arena and in their broader lives. The Curriculum-Based Training method not only amplifies performance but also fosters the personal evolution and advancement of young swimmers, positioning them for success in the competitive realm of swimming and beyond.

With a strong emphasis on holistic skill development, equitable time management across all racing disciplines, prevention of over-specialization, psychological well-being, strategic planning, and goal-setting, Curriculum-Based Training offers a comprehensive framework to enhance young swimmers' love for competitive swimming.

Utilizing a deliberate practice methodology and the spiral curriculum model, swimmers have the opportunity to systematically improve their skills and mental fortitude. By creating an environment that mirrors competitive conditions, and by implementing structured training that encompasses warm-ups, training sets, and relays, young swimmers are empowered to maximize their experience in the sport of swimming. Such a holistic approach not only cultivates technical excellence but also nurtures valuable life skills, including discipline, resilience, and a collaborative spirit.

In conclusion, the Curriculum-Based Training approach provides a comprehensive and efficient training program designed to equip young swimmers for success in competitive swimming. Its structured framework facilitates collaboration between coaches and swimmers to establish a solid foundation for skill enhancement, goal attainment, and overall proficiency in the sport.

By emphasizing targeted skill enhancement through deliberate practice, reinforcing fundamental skills via the spiral curriculum model, and fostering proficiency in skill acquisition using the blocked practice principle, young swimmers are steadily prepared for success both in the pool and, more generally, in life. Deliberate practice facilitates a structured and systematic skill development process, the spiral curriculum model promotes continuous learning and mastery, and the blocked practice principle improves skill retention and proficiency. Through the incorporation of psychological strategies, Curriculum-Based Training also addresses issues such as performance anxiety, peer pressure, and motivation, ultimately resulting in long-term benefits. These include aspects such as increased resilience, enhanced focus, sustained motivation, improved self-efficacy, cultivation of a growth mindset, enhanced coping mechanisms, stress management, and lasting performance improvement. The Curriculum-Based Training approach propels young swimmers towards comprehensive growth and achievement in competitive swimming and beyond.

Looking to the Future

The knowledge described in this book serves as a foundation for further development of the training approaches used in swimming. Coaches, athletes, and parents are encouraged to adopt Curriculum-Based Training as a new way of thinking for young swimmers and their preparation for training and competitions. Through increased intentional learning, gradual progression, and encouraging cooperation, future generations of swimmers will be enabled to reach their full potential.

To support the implementation and refinement of Curriculum-Based Training, future books will delve deeper into specific aspects of this approach, including:

- "Implementing Curriculum-Based Training for Young Swimmers"
- "Developing Competitive Swimming Strokes through Curriculum-Based Training"
- "The Psychology of Curriculum-Based Training in Competitive Swimming"

Curriculum-Based Training is a young swimmers' program aimed at the development of skills, mastering them, and proceeding to competition. The program uses Bruner's spiral curriculum and Ericsson's deliberate practice approach and provides a clear framework for how abilities can be developed and how a person can achieve mastery in the pool. From the conception of the stroke to the final competition stage, the Curriculum-Based Training system is based on gradual skill improvement, psychological preparation, the definition of goals, and team assistance. Young swimmers are prepared for competitive swimming through the use of consistent practice structures and an emphasis on specific skill development.

Adopting Curriculum-Based Training values encourages positive behavior and progress within the sporting organization, and assists young swimmers to attain their competitive objectives and acquire relevant skills for a lifetime. It's time to take the first step with confidence, with purpose, and to aim for— and achieve—the highest standards.

ABOUT THE AUTHOR

Rapolas Janonis, affectionately known as Coach Rap, is a remarkable first-time author whose profound background in competitive swimming and coaching has shaped his unique approach to holistic athlete development. Born in Soviet Union-era Lithuania, Coach Rap began his journey in competitive swimming at a young age, representing his country on the international stage before moving to the United States for his collegiate swimming career. His endeavors led to notable achievements, including pioneering the SWIM RIGHT Method, solidifying his place as an inspiring figure in the swimming community.

With a master's degree in kinesiology, Coach Rap has delved deeply into the principles of specificity and sports psychology, shaping his coaching philosophy. He has dedicated nearly two decades to researching and analyzing young swimmers' performances. Drawing on the extensive research of acclaimed theorists like Dr. Jerome S. Bruner and Dr. Anders Ericsson, Coach Rap has masterfully developed a revolutionary Curriculum-Based Training method that maximizes the unique talents of every young swimmer.

REFERENCES

Adam, J. (n.d.). "Improve Your Swimming by Using Zones: A Beginner's Guide." Retrieved May 27, 2024. https://www.trainingpeaks.com/blog/a-beginners-guide-to-swim-training/

Busch, B. (2024, May 9). "Deliberate practice: What separates Elite Athletes from the rest." InnerDrive. https://www.innerdrive.co.uk/blog/deliberate-practice-athletes/

Clear, J. (n.d.). "Deliberate Practice: What It Is and How to Use It." James Clear.com. Retrieved May 27, 2024. https://jamesclear.com/deliberate-practice-theory#:~:text=Deliberate%20practice%20refers%20to%20a,specific%20goal%20of%20improving%20performance.

Donnelly, J. (2020, January 31). "Examining risks, benefits, and how coaches can guide athletes." Coach and Athletic Director. https://coachad.com/articles/sport-specialization-risks-benefits/

Dweck, C. (2016, January 13). "What Having a "Growth Mindset" Actually Means." Harvard Business Review. Retrieved May 27, 2024. https://hbr.org/2016/01/what-having-a-growth-mindset-actually-means

Haugen, T., & Seiler, S. (2019, November 21). "The training and development of Elite Sprint Performance: An integration of scientific and best practice literature." Sports Medicine - Open. SpringerOpen. https://sportsmedicine-open.springeropen.com/articles/10.1186/s40798-019-0221-0

Kenny, K. (2023, August 25). "Teaching Swimming Lessons with a Growth Mindset Approach: Enhancing Skill Acquisition and Psychological Resilience." Retrieved May 27, 2024, from https://onewiththewater.org/teaching-swimming-lessons-growth-mindset-psychological-resilience/

Kucera, T. (2024, April 7). "Deliberate Practice Explained: How Focused Training Transforms Skill Acquisition." The Geeky Leader.com. Retrieved May 27, 2024. https://thegeekyleader.com/2024/04/07/deliberate-practice-explained-how-focused-training-transforms-skill-acquisition/#:~:text=It%20involves%20engaging%20in%20activities,specific%20goal%20of%20improving%20performance.

Main, P. (2022, January 6). "The Spiral Curriculum: A Teacher's Guide." Structural learning.com. Retrieved May 27, 2024. https://www.structural-learning.com/post/the-spiral-curriculum-a-teachers-guide

Reeves, M. (2024, April 15). "A Detailed Guide to Skills-Based Training." Together Platform.com. Retrieved May 27, 2024. https://www.togetherplatform.com/blog/skills-based-training

RLS. (n.d.). "It's Time to Thrive with Swim and Survive." Royal Life Sving.com. Retrieved May 27, 2024. https://www.royallifesaving.com.au/educate-participate/swimming/swim-and-survive

Salo, Dave. Ph.D. (1989). Sprint Salo (pdf). Sports Support Syndicate, inc. Retrieved May 27, 2024. https://www.teamunify.com/tsc/__doc__/146380_4_Sprintsalo.pdf

SL. (2023, May 3). "Jerome Bruner's Theories." Structural learning.com. Retrieved May 27, 2024. https://www.structural-learning.com/post/jerome-bruners-theories#:~:text=The%20Spiral%20Curriculum%3A%0A%20Unique,building%20upon%20previously%20learned%20concepts.

SM. (2024, May 15). "Swimming Mental Training: Techniques For Maintaining Motivation And Managing Pressure." Swim Mirror.com. Retrieved May 27, 2024. https://swimmirror.com/blog/swimming-mental-training-techniques-for-maintaining-motivation-and-managing-pressure/#:~:text=Techniques%20such%20as%20goal%20setting,their%20success%20as%20physical%20training.